How to Permanently Cure Your Fear of Public Speaking

LISA BAUM

How to Permanently Cure Your Fear of Public Speaking

Published by Wheatmark™
610 East Delano Street, Suite 104, Tucson, Arizona 85705
U.S.A.
www.wheatmark.com

ISBN-13: 978-1-58736-739-7
ISBN-10: 1-58736-739-4
LCCN: 2006939471

Acknowledgments

I want to thank my Lord and Savior Jesus Christ who has given me true life, hope, meaning, purpose, contentment and the ability to just accept myself for who I am. Jesus has brought me to a place in my life that I never thought I would ever be able to reach and He has enabled me to accomplish and become more than I ever thought I could.

I would also like to thank my twin brother Andy who means more to me than words could possibly express. Andy has been to me a father, mother, personal trainer, life coach, encourager and my best friend and I just wanted to let him know how much I love him and how very proud I am of him and the person he has become and what he has accomplished in his life. Andy's words and wisdom have helped me greatly over the years to believe in myself and to make better decisions and I love him very much! I also would like to tell my husband Vance that he is the one and only love of my life (and believe me one is enough!), To Mom, Dad, Casey and Kristy and Joggy I love each of you very much and I am grateful to have you all in my life.

Contents

Introduction

This book is not a collection of tricks and techniques for a quick fix to your public speaking fears and phobias. This book is all about getting to the root causes of your public speaking fears and getting rid of them permanently. I truly believe that the truths within this book will help you to "Permanently Cure Your Fear of Public Speaking". I have seen from my own life experiences that public speaking fears and phobias are simply the results of a poor self image. As we move further along I will identify and explain this in more detail and define this more specifically as low self esteem and low self confidence and the fear of man. I believe that the simple truths within these pages will help you to truly be free to speak in public and just be yourself. Conquering your fears and phobias of public speaking will not only help you to become a better speaker but will also greatly impact every other area of your life as well. You will not experience those fears and anxiety's anymore as you face public speaking situations or any type of social situation for that matter because you will become a genuinely more confident person and it all starts with knowing that you are exactly the same as everyone else and that you have the exact same value as everyone else.

If you are serious about overcoming your public speaking fears, anxieties and phobias and you choose to move forward and deal with the root causes of low self esteem and low self confidence in your life, you will eventually come to realize that there is nothing to fear about public speaking if you really know your true value.

I start off this book by sharing a little bit about myself and my childhood so you can understand a few things about me and how I developed my poor self image and faulty belief system which has caused me to fear speaking in public all of my life. Through sharing my experiences I lay a foundation for a few concepts that I will explain in detail later on, but regardless of the type of childhood or life experiences you have had, I identify three key areas that I believe all public speaking fears can be traced back to and I truly believe will help you to help yourself to overcome this embarrassing problem once and for all.

Painful Childhood Experiences

My dad was an alcoholic and beat me and my brother several times a day with "the strap". I am now almost 38 years old and I still remember what this strap looked like and the memories of these beatings and the settings in which they took place. My brother and I have had many very painful and traumatic experiences growing up because of my father's alcohol and abuse as well as being children of and witnesses to a very painful and ugly divorce. Most of us have had or known others who have had very painful childhood experiences and very painful life experiences for that matter so this is nothing new, but fact is whether we want to admit it or not these traumatic experiences have shaped our beliefs and perceptions of ourselves and the world around us and still affects most of us today in one way or another. I developed beliefs and perceptions about myself that I had little value because I perceived the beatings I received from my father as "I must not have any value and I must not be worthy of love or I would not be beaten like this". So I grew up facing life with these unhealthy and distorted beliefs and perceptions about myself and dragging my emotional pain and hang-ups with me along the way. But I have reached the point in my life where I am tired of feeling like a worthless piece of garbage because of what I have learned to believe about myself and the bottom line is that even though these painful experiences happened to me I must take responsibility for my life and correct these perceptions of myself in order to enjoy and succeed in life. It is up to each one of us to decide if we will choose to move forward into our future no matter what has happened to us. We all need to decide if we were going to continue blaming the people and experiences of our past that have caused us a lot of pain and helped us to form our faulty self perceptions and poor self image or to take responsibility for the fact that we have allowed the way other people have treated us to cause us low self esteem and low self confidence by believing that the treatment we received was somehow our fault or that we deserved it in some way instead of realizing that it was those who inflicted pain upon us who had the real problems not us.

My twin brother and I were beaten by our alcoholic father throughout our childhood. My father abused us both physically and verbally until we were about five years old and then my parents divorced. After my parents divorced my dad would disappear for months and years at a time. The abuse we received as children was instrumental in the way both my brother and I learned to perceive ourselves and our childhood experiences were the foundation that our negative beliefs and poor self image were built upon and have hindered us most of our lives.

Poor self image, low self esteem, and not believing in myself were some of the negative beliefs that I had. These beliefs were created by the way I perceived my value as I went through the abuse I experienced growing up. I became exactly what I believed I was, a person who had no value, unlovable, depressed and struggling through each day instead of enjoying and experiencing life. I saw myself as one that had no value and lived out exactly what I believed of myself and my beliefs became my reality. I believed I was not capable of achieving much and felt like I had very little value because of the self perceptions that I formed as a child.

Self Image Must Change

After some serious soul searching, I came to the conclusion that I needed to change my self image because It was no longer my childhood holding me back, it was now me holding me back by continuing to believe those lies and warped perceptions of myself that I had formed while growing up. The key to breaking out of those unhealthy perceptions of low self esteem and low self confidence was transforming my mind and belief system by God's Word, the Bible. Just as my negative beliefs and expectations were the key factors in creating a life far less than I was capable of combined with depression and fears, my positive beliefs and expectations of myself have enabled me to create a life for myself that is full of hopes, dreams and goals and the ability to believe in myself. Whatever we believe and expect of ourselves will become our reality. We can harness this power of belief to create a life of success or we can use this same power to create a life of defeat, the choice is up to us. Just as we use anti-virus software on our computers to rid them of deadly electronic viruses that can cripple our hard drives, we must take the same type of corrective action in combating our negative thoughts, beliefs and perceptions which cripple us in our minds and hearts, at the very core of our beings. A great biblical example of how poor self image and warped perceptions stop us from succeeding and moving forward in our lives is from the book of Numbers 13:31-33 (Chapter 13, Verse 31-33), basically what happens in this chapter is that the Lord commands Moses to send out one man from every tribe of the children of Israel to go and check out the land that God has promised to give them as their inheritance. Verse 31 tells us that these men brought back a negative report to Moses as follows "But the men that went up with them said we are not able to go up against the people of the land for they are stronger than we are". Verse 32 these men say "…the land looks like it swallows up its inhabitants and the people we saw there are men of great stature". Verse 33 states "And we saw the giants, the sons of Anak which come from the giants and we were in our own sight as grasshoppers and so we were also in their sight". So to sum up these verses, these men show us how our faulty beliefs, distorted perceptions and the fear man hinder us from claiming what is rightfully ours. These men had poor self images and because of this they perceived themselves as inferior to the natives of the land that they were spying out. These men also wrongly perceived and jumped to false conclusions about what the natives of the land thought about them as they were spying out the land and sad to say these ten men never entered into their promised land, they died in a barren and dry wilderness. Two of these men however did believe in God's promise and also believed in themselves and their abilities and they did go up to possess the Promised Land and lived very successful and fruitful lives. My point to all of this is to show you how our warped perceptions, low self esteem and basically just a poor self image will stop us from moving forward into our future and our destiny. Our perceptions, low self esteem, low self confidence and the fear of man will taint everything we experience in life and cause us to not only believe lies about ourselves and our abilities but will also cause us to incorrectly assume and jump to the wrong conclusions about what other people think about us. *The Bible says in II Corinthians 10:5 "Casting down imaginations, and every high thing that exalteth itself against the knowledge of God, and bringing into captivity every thought to the obedience of Christ".* We are told in the Bible how important it is to think properly and if a thought that you have is contrary to what God has said about you than you need to throw it away.

Nothing will ever change in our lives until we become determined to change our perceptions and beliefs of ourselves and the world around us. Even though I was not the cause of the abuse I received from my father, I am responsible as an adult for continuing to allow it to affect me. It was my choice to no longer allow the negative perceptions that I have had of myself to control my future. If I wanted to achieve the goals I had deep within my heart and reach my full potential as a human being, I had to take the responsibility of changing the way I saw myself in order to become the person I wanted to be, the person I knew I really was deep down inside.

The way out of my self defeating beliefs was creating new, healthy, realistic and truthful thoughts and perceptions of myself. It has taken me most of my adult life learning how to undo the damage that had been done to my self-image and I am still learning. Today I am no longer held captive by who I thought I was. I am in the process of being transformed from the inside out by choosing to think and believe differently about myself. I have by no means been perfected in this area, but I have made great progress and I am encouraged by all of the successes along the way. Each time I accomplish something, I get strengthened with the courage and self-confidence to keep moving forward, to keep learning and growing and to never stop trying to accomplish my goals.

My journey of self discovery and growth has been full of challenges. I have had to challenge myself to embrace new images and expectations of myself and to believe in myself even though it was contrary to all that ever I knew. Little by little, replacing one negative thought and belief at a time my life has been changed. I am no longer seeing myself as the hopeless, unlovely, worthless person I believed I once was. I now know that there is great power when I believe in myself and have faith in God. It is exciting to be able to see the truth about who I really am and being able to uncover the lies and negative thinking patterns of the past has been very liberating.

Learning Healthy Beliefs and Perceptions

As I mentioned, I have been involved in an on-going process of replacing those old negative beliefs and the poor self image that I have had of myself with positive, loving, healthy beliefs and the change in my life and my attitude is really amazing. My inner world and my mind have changed in very positive ways enabling me to move forward in my life and achieve my goals. I have a fresh new view of myself and I am a much more positive person. I am now able to believe in myself and all of the possibilities of what I can become in this life.

Once I set goals of what I wanted to accomplish and the type of person I wanted to become I really saw great changes happen. As soon as I made the decision to move forward toward my goals of reaching my full potential as a human being, I stepped out in faith with positive beliefs and expectations and the details have seemed to work themselves out in truly amazing ways with God's help. It is amazing to see how each decision for positive change just builds upon itself and each step forward toward those changes builds momentum and my future keeps getting brighter and brighter as I step out and keep walking towards my goals and dreams not allowing those lies of the past to keep me in darkness anymore.

We as human beings have power, more power than we realize. We have the power to choose, to make decisions, and the power to control our thoughts, beliefs and emotions. Being in control of ourselves is really the key to living a successful and fulfilling life. We cannot control other people or many of our circumstances in life but we can certainly learn to control ourselves if we have the desire and willingness to learn. We must be hopeful and think upon things that are true and things that will build us up, not tear us down, even the Bible states this in Philippians 4:8 (Chapter 4, Verse 8) *"Finally brethren, whatever is true, whatever is honorable, whatever is right, whatever is pure, whatever is lovely, whatever is of good repute, if there is any excellence and if anything worthy of praise, let your mind dwell on these things"*.

I am very encouraged by the successes in my life so far and I know I will be learning new skills of self empowerment for the rest of my life. Please understand that I am by no means suggesting that if you just think positively and think good thoughts that everything will be alright and you will receive everything you hope for and life will be great, I am not saying that at all. I do not agree at all with any type of teaching where people believe they can create realities with their minds. This type of teaching is very dangerous and not in accordance with reality. What I am saying is that we need to believe and think about ourselves in a healthy way, accurately, soberly and correctly in order to rebuild our self esteem and self confidence in those areas that cause us to experience the symptoms of fear and anxiety when we have to speak in public.

Whatever we hope to achieve in our lives one thing is certain whatever we believe we can or cannot do will be true for us. When we believe in ourselves and God it seems like all things are possible and a new world of possibilities opens up to us. Jesus even states in the book of *Mark 9:23 (Chapter 9, Verse 23): "All things are possible to him who believes"*. Our attitudes and thoughts create our perceptions of ourselves and pave the road to our destiny. We must constantly strive to see our lives, other people and our circumstances as opportunities to grow and learn if we have the desire to change. We must learn to develop a more healthy and positive view of ourselves and to look for the good in our daily lives and count our blessings. Yes there are failures, disappointments and suffering in this life but we must somehow look for that silver lining and try to find the good in a situation even though it may be very difficult at times. We cannot control many of the circumstances in our lives but we can learn to perceive them in a different way in order to be able to get through them and to learn from them and grow from them. Our beliefs and thoughts create a very pleasant internal environment within our hearts and minds which help us to deal with very unpleasant external circumstances that life sometimes brings us.

Whatever we believe about ourselves will be our lot in life. Our beliefs have power and it is our beliefs that build the foundation that our lives are built upon. It is our beliefs that cause us to be secure in who we are at the very core of our being. Our beliefs strengthen us and build us up and it is our beliefs about ourselves that make us feel confident and valuable and secure, therefore we must make a greater effort to develop healthy perceptions and beliefs about ourselves. We must make an honest assessment of ourselves and try to see areas in our lives that have been hindered due to our low self esteem and poor self image because it is these faulty beliefs that we have about ourselves that are the root causes of why we fear speaking in public. I don't really believe that any of us actually have the fear public speaking, I believe it is our low self esteem and low self confidence and not understanding our true value that causes us to fear speaking to an audience. Therefore we must be willing to let go of our negative belief system and we must choose to embrace the truth about who we are and it all starts with our beliefs about who we are and how we perceive ourselves.

Real Change Comes
from Within

My conclusion is that all change in our lives must start from the inside out. The world today is constantly looking for the next new thing that will help us feel better about ourselves externally, extreme makeovers, plastic surgery and new trends, stylish clothing in the hottest colors and special moisturizers that promise to fill in our wrinkles and even out our skin tone. I like all of those things I just mentioned, I have no problem with any of that stuff, we all want to look and feel great including myself. What I am trying to say is that you can have all of those things that I just mentioned and look marvelous on the outside but those things will not fix the real you which is the internal part of you, your inner man. The real you that lives inside that body that possess all of those external things. It is our belief system and expectations about ourselves that affect our behavior and how we view ourselves and the world around us.

Before we can take action to change we must have a plan and set realistic goals for ourselves and before we have a plan, we must have healthy beliefs and expectations of ourselves in order to make our plans a reality. If we care about where we are headed on this journey of life we must be honest with ourselves and ask ourselves if we are where we would like to be or if we are at least taking the necessary action to get ourselves headed down the right path. Each one of us is responsible for our own happiness and success. If we are not successful or fulfilled or finding joy in our daily lives we have no one to blame but ourselves. We are in charge of ourselves and we are responsible for the decisions we make. If we care at all about our future we must take the corrective action necessary to make our beliefs and expectations more positive and healthy. We must learn to accept ourselves and others just as we are while constantly striving to learn and grow and become the people we know deep down inside of our hearts we know we can be.

The bottom line is we all need to "just get over it and move on" and the "it" in that phrase is whatever "it" is that is holding you back from moving forward with your life so it is up to you to fill in that blank. While it is true that we all do need to "just get over it" most people that have experienced such painful childhood and life experiences have become such emotional and mental cripples in certain areas of their lives that they just can't "get over it" at the snap of one's fingers, some of these damaged souls like myself have had to go through major counseling and a lot of pain in facing and confronting our issues and had to work very hard at "getting over it", it just takes desire and effort. We all know people or have heard stories about others who have overcome great hardships in their lives and have gone on to become great successes so we know it is certainly possible it just depends on how much effort we put into overcoming our issues whatever they may be.

Life is short and seems to be moving by faster and

faster everyday and you and I have all wasted enough time lamenting over our past hurts and disappointments and crying in our soup, so it is time for each of us to live our lives before our lives are over in order to make sure we don't have any regret about "what could have been". I know many adults who still talk about painful childhood memories that happened over 20 or 30 years ago and they can either continue to re-live those painful experiences in their minds and talk about them all of the time and choose to hang on to all that junk or get just accept it and get rid of it and move on, it's up to them. Nothing good will ever come from carrying around all that extra baggage of hurts and hang-ups and pain and insecurity, it does nothing but weigh us down, make us depressed and stop us from living and enjoying life and becoming all we can be. *The Book of Hebrews 12:1 (Chapter 12, Verse 1) states "...let us lay aside every weight, and the sin which doth so easily beset us, and let us run with patience the race that is set before us"*. We are told to lay aside every weight that we are carrying; this weight represents those things that hinder us from continuing on our journey of life successfully.

Public Speaking Fears, Anxicties, and Phobias

But to get back to my story I can't remember exactly when all of my fears started but what I do know is that I have lived with so many different types of ridiculous and irrational fears, phobias and anxieties most of my life due to what I believe all come from my low self esteem and low self confidence and how I have allowed my past experiences and childhood to make me feel about myself.

What I am going to focus on in this book is my own public speaking phobia. Growing up I was the one in class that would rather take a failing grade instead of getting up in front of the class to do an oral report as I am sure many of you are. I just continued on in my life avoiding speaking situations at all costs. As I advanced on in my career life I realized that at any given time I could be called upon at a moment's notice to walk into a meeting and actively participate or speak to a group because it was happening all around me. When I saw it happening to my co-workers my heart would race and I would have an anxiety attack right at my desk at even the thought that this could happen to me. But as time went on and the older I got I realized that these fears of public speaking would never go away until I made a choice to confront them and somehow overcome them so I decided to join Toastmasters at the suggestion of someone I had met in order to help myself work through my fears of public speaking and also to get some practice and experience speaking in front of a group. My participation in Toastmasters caused me to really want to find out the reasons "why" I have had these paralyzing fears of public speaking my whole life and the whole package of hang-ups that comes with it, the anxiety, sweats, chills, heart palpitations, being overly self-conscious and all of the terrifying thoughts and feelings of facing the moment when you have to get up and speak to an audience. What I discovered about myself was that public speaking was not the real problem even though I thought it was, it was only the result of my real problems which I have discovered to be low self esteem, low self confidence and the fear of man. Discovering these three things about myself has really changed my life. I have finally identified the true causes of why I have struggled with public speaking fears and phobias all of my life and because of this I am able to deal with the real source of the problem and correct it and move forward with my life.

I know that each one of us has our own unique set of fears, anxieties and hang-ups about public speaking but I am convinced that these symptoms can all be traced back to these three issues that I have already mentioned. It is not about learning techniques, tricks or tips in order to "control" these horrible symptoms such as the crippling fears, the anxiety, panic attacks, heart palpitations, throwing up, knees knocking, light headedness and dizziness which are not only degrading but make people who struggle with low self esteem and low self confidence and a poor self image feel even worse about themselves and even more embarrassed. I have experienced most of these symptoms myself and for those of us that already struggle with low self esteem and low self confidence we certainly don't need anything else to make us feel worse about ourselves, right?

The purpose of this book is to encourage each of you to deal with the root causes of your public speaking fears in your own lives and hearts in order to be permanently cured from the fear of public speaking. Once you deal with the real issues causing you to fear public speaking you will be able to stand up and speak to your audience free from all fear and confident in who you are and you will be comfortable in just being yourself in front of your audience. If you truly desire to win your public speaking battle it is up to you to reflect on some of your own faulty beliefs and perceptions of yourself and then correct them by developing healthy beliefs and perceptions about yourself in these areas that I have just described.

Confronting Three Key Areas Will Help You to Speak Without Fear

I believe that these three key areas that I have discovered about myself are all somehow related and I'll tell you why. If you have low self esteem you don't have a good opinion of yourself or feel that you have any value and because you don't believe that you have any value you don't have much self confidence which then causes you to be fearful of speaking to other people or groups of people because you somehow believe that you are lower or less important than others which makes you feel anxious and fearful knowing that you have to speak to other people whom you believe to be so much better than you are or somehow higher than you are which then causes you more anxiety and fear about what they might think of you. Uncovering this ridiculous spiral of beliefs and perceptions has made a huge difference in my life. I finally realized that my fears and phobias about public speaking were all just symptoms of my real problems which were my poor self image and how I perceived my own self worth. My childhood abuse and painful life experiences caused me to view other people as so much better than I was and that I was so much lower than they were and this I believe was the root cause of all my public speaking phobias.

So to recap, I have discovered three key areas about myself that have caused my public speaking fears:

1. Low Self Esteem
2. Low Self Confidence
3. The Fear of Man

We will take a deeper look at each of these in just a moment but first I want to say that this book is not about teaching you a few cool techniques or tricks that you can just apply externally to your public speaking situation. "How to Permanently Cure Your Fear of Public Speaking" gets to the heart of the matter, literally. This book focuses on the beliefs in your heart and the way you perceive yourself and how to truly develop genuine self esteem and self confidence. I say genuine because when something is genuine it is real and authentic it is not some trick or technique that you have to learn and practice and it is not about spending thousands of dollars to travel to a special seminar or conference in some other part of the country to learn a few techniques, it is about real and permanent change inside of your heart. It is about learning that you have value and just as much value as every other human being in the world whether rich or poor, black or white, etc., we are all equal and have equal value. The value that I am talking about is the value that we possess simply because God created all of us equal and therefore we no longer have to view others as better than we are because it just simply is not true. Strip away the big corporate titles, the big bank accounts, the fancy and expensive suits and big houses;

I am not talking about this kind of external value. The value that I keep talking about is the value that we all possess as human beings. There are plenty of quick fixes out there that promise change but you and I both know and have probably tried many of these types of quick fixes in our lives over the years and they just don't work or produce the permanent results were are looking for and then we just go on looking for the next thing that promises to help us.

I have really been able to move forward with my life not avoiding meetings, social situations or speaking opportunities but I am now ready if an opportunity should present itself because my beliefs in my heart have changed and I have learned my true value and I have gained true self confidence and true self esteem and no one or nothing can take that away from me no matter what life may bring. My goal in life is not to be the best speaker in the world because I have no desire to be nor am I trying to be. My goal is just to be confident, comfortable and at peace if and when the time comes where I do need to get up and speak to a group, make a presentation of some kind, actively participate in a meeting or go on a job interview. Today I can stand at the podium and deliver a twelve minute speech but if you could have seen me a while back I could not even stand in front of a group of people, much less speak to them. I am very proud of myself and grateful to God for the progress that I have made. I feel like a huge obstacle in my life has now been removed and it is a great feeling to finally be on the other side of this problem for this first time in my life.

Low Self Esteem

I looked up the word esteem in the dictionary and some of the definitions given were value, worth, and opinion. So, if you have low self esteem it means that you have a low opinion of yourself and that you do not value yourself. Healthy self esteem means the exact opposite. It means you have a healthy opinion of yourself and that you value yourself not in a haughty or arrogant or obnoxious way but in a way that is healthy and real and true and comes from knowing that every human being has the exact same value regardless of what they do for a living or how much money they make or their education level. True and healthy beliefs will enable you to be genuinely comfortable and at peace speaking in front of anyone at anytime without fear. The key is knowing and understanding that all human beings are created equal and are of equal value not because of what they do for a living or what they have or what they look like but because God has created all of us equal and has bestowed upon us great value and dignity as human beings. So when you are facing a group that you must speak to you must realize that everyone else in the room has the same exact value as you do regardless of what their title or position is in the company, etc. If you have low self esteem you are unable to see your own value and right to dignity as a human being and you will have great fear and anxiety as you speak to others because you don't feel like you have any worth or that you are not as good as others and because of this you have no self confidence in expressing yourself because you somehow view others as better or somehow higher than you are and that is simply not true.

Low Self Confidence

I also looked up the word confidence in the dictionary and one of the definitions given was to be certain. So if you are certain of yourself and of who you are and your abilities you will be able to express yourself confidently to others without faking it or getting nervous because you have nothing to prove and you can just be yourself. It is not about covering something up or learning a quick technique to help you through a public speaking situation it is about real and permanent change by curing the unhealthy beliefs and perceptions that you have about yourself and others and there is a world of difference between these two solutions. It is about being truly certain and sure of yourself deep within your heart about your value and abilities no matter what situation you find yourself in. You will never have any reason to be anxious or nervous in front of anyone or in any type of social situation for that matter because we are all equal we are all the same and we are all human and that is the reason why none of us are better than anyone else. Yes we all look different and dress differently and earn different salaries and have different talents and abilities that is true but I am not talking about these types of external things. I am talking about looking upon yourself and others not by these external things but by our humanity our common characteristics as human beings which is what makes us all the same. We are all flesh and blood and it is these human characteristics that help us to see that at the very core of our beings after all the outward stuff is stripped away we are all the same and that alone should help you to realize there is absolutely nothing to fear about speaking to a group of people who are exactly like you, human! I do have to say that not everyone thinks like this, most people walk around thinking and acting like they are so much better than everyone else and they are truly wrong and deceived even delusional and impressed with their own unimportance (my dad used to say that). I also believe that these people have low self esteem and low self confidence as well because these types of arrogant and haughty people are trying to cover up their beliefs and perceptions about themselves by going to the other extreme and exalting themselves over others. Both extremes are wrong and need to be corrected in order to be free of the anxiety's and fears of public speaking.

The Fear of Man

The Bible says in Proverbs 29:25 (chapter 29, verse 25)
"the fear of man brings a snare" (which is a trap, some-
thing that someone can get entangled in or ensnared by). I
was caught up in this trap for most of my life and I feel
great freedom in my life now because I finally realized
that I don't need to fear what other people think of me
because whatever they think of me really doesn't matter anyway. The opinions of others are not important in
life unless you ask for them but even if you don't ask
there are some people that must give you their opinion
anyway. It is not my concern what people think of me, I
don't have to answer to them and my life is none of their
business. They don't pay my bills and their opinions of
me have no impact on my life, they are just like me and
it really doesn't matter what they think of me anyway. I
don't owe people anything except the respect that is due
to each of us as we interact with our fellow man.

We all share the same human nature and we are all
born with this need or desire to be liked, loved, accepted and well thought of by others. This is a beautiful
thought but the reality is not everyone is going to love us
or even like us and some will even hate us and that's just
how it is. I have seen many people go to great lengths

to try to impress others or look good in front of others in order to be accepted or somehow well thought of by others, even other people that they don't know (how ridiculous is that?). Why not just be yourself and just live your life and give up trying to make a good impression on people because if people are going to like you, it is the real "you" that they are going to like anyway not some phony version of yourself that you are trying pass off as real and besides even if they don't like you who cares anyway, they are no better than you are and your life's mission should be to be the best "you" you can be it should not be trying to please other people and you and I both know there are some people that will never be pleased not matter what you do. Most people are fickle they are fond of you one minute and the moment you make a mistake or say something they don't like or when they no longer have a need for you then they don't like you anymore so why bother, forget it and move forward with your life by being free from the fear of caring about what others think of you. For some reason we all try to put on some type of outward show in front of others because deep down we all want to be liked, loved, accepted and look good in front of others and it is just a big waste of time, emotional energy and it is also very draining and distracting from your goals and responsibilities in life.

Just Be Yourself

For some reason people are just not comfortable and at peace with just being themselves. Yes, it's that simple, just be yourself. My brother has often repeated this to me many times over the years and he was right. Being yourself takes all of the pressure off of you to "perform" or "act" in a certain way or try to be someone or something you are not in speaking situations or social situations. It is very sad that our society has been brainwashed into thinking this way probably because people are just simply afraid to just be who they really are because most people really don't know who they really are or feel secure in who they are anyway which is why they are putting on an outward show in the first place. People know when they see something real or not, say for example, you are in a meeting and you are asked a question that you do not have an answer to at that particular moment it is perfectly ok to say "I am sorry I don't have an answer for you right now but I would be happy to find out for you and get back to you a little bit later". Most people are afraid to be honest with others and are unable to say those three horrible words "I don't know", because they fear what other people think about them than instead of just being real and honest and just being themselves.

You have probably heard that slang phrase that has been used quite a bit in our society among the young people, they say "keep it real", well this is very good advice just keep it real. I have seen many people in similar types of situations in my life while attending meetings and in my opinion I think most people feel like they must have an answer for everything and would never really want to be honest and say "I don't know" because they are trying to prove somehow that they have it altogether and that they are somehow more important and more intelligent than others in the room and they want to be perceived as better than others or smarter than others. I believe that these people have low self esteem and low self confidence also because they fear what other people will think about them at that moment and because they do not genuinely feel good about just being themselves or comfortable in just being who they are they try to put on some kind of show and it really turns out to be a freak show of pride and ego's and arrogant and controlling behavior. It is very sad but also very ugly and pathetic at the same time.

People who are insecure and have low self esteem and low self confidence do either one of two things, they either view themselves as inferior to other people or the exact opposite they see themselves as being so much better than others and both views are completely unbalanced and wrong and will cause great fear in public speaking situations. "Just be yourself" are truly great words of wisdom but if you don't know your true value or don't believe you have much value it is impossible to just rest and be at peace with who you are and to "just be yourself". Meetings, public speaking and social events would be so much more enjoyable if we could all just be ourselves. No striving to make a good impression no putting on false fronts or outward shows for others but just being comfortable in being who we truly are. WOW! Could you just imagine how much more fun and enjoyable meetings and social events would be and how much more could be accomplished at business meetings if we could just be ourselves not competing with others but coming together with others to just brainstorm and exchange ideas and have discussions without the ego's, pride, manipulating, obnoxious and arrogant control freaks who need to try to prove and somehow show everyone how important and intelligent they are. The truth is most people will not change, but we must change in order to accomplish our goals and live our lives in the beautiful freedom that God has provided.

We Are Equally Valuable

The fact is we are all equally important. We are all intelligent in different ways but the problem is that most people think they are the only one's that are important and intelligent and that everyone else is so much less than they are but they are just legends in their own minds. We are all equally important and equally valuable not because of the status we have attained in this life or the wealth we have accumulated but because we are all human, one race of people, human beings with intelligence and value because the Bible says in *Psalm 139:14 (Psalm 139, verse 14) "we are all fearfully (awesome) and wonderfully made"*. Our bodies, our organs, our brains and the miracle of our eyes which give us sight, our blood and how our bodies were created, it is truly amazing, think about that for a while and then think about the fact that even though we all look different and have different talents and abilities we all share the exact same humanity.

These simple truths have helped me so much in my life to realize that we are all equal and I have nothing to fear anymore about speaking in public. Those lies of my past are gone and these truths have come and set me free from all that garbage of warped and skewed perceptions of myself. One of my favorite Bible verses is very appropriate here, in *John 8:32 (Chapter 8, Verse 32) Jesus states, "You shall know the truth and the truth shall make you free"*. The bottom line is our childhood's and painful life experiences and how we have allowed those experiences to make us feel have somehow taught us to believe lies about ourselves and what all of us need to do is just replace those lies with the truth and we will finally be free. That is why I said earlier that this book is not about tricks and techniques; it is about permanent and lasting change by developing healthy and genuine self esteem and self confidence. These are the real keys to change and they will enable you to truly be able to speak without fear and will not only make you a better and more confident speaker but will make you a more successful person in life and that's what it's all about.

Transforming Your Mind

There are zillions of self help books out there that give you quick fixes on how to change your behavior or give you a few techniques to overcome a situation but I am convinced from my own life experiences that it is not our behavior that needs modification, it is the way we see and perceive ourselves, our value and others that is the real problem. Many in the mental health profession think they have discovered the true answer to real change and they have called it "reprogramming". However the Bible told us this exact same thing almost two thousand years ago, sometime around 56 – 58 AD to be exact. *The Bible says in Romans 12:2 (Chapter 12, verse 2) "...Be transformed by the renewing of your mind".* Our minds and hearts need to be renewed and transformed from our negative beliefs, perceptions and poor self images which keep us down and depressed and hopeless and then and only then will our behavior change it is not the other way around.

My whole life I have learned to see myself as having no value because that is what I learned and perceived from my experiences growing up. It takes time to unlearn the skewed and warped perceptions and unhealthy beliefs about yourself and to learn true and healthy ways of thinking and believing about yourself and others. No matter how you have been treated or what types of circumstances you have been through, we are all equal even though you might not feel that way. I am not sure exactly who said it but I love this expression "there is level ground at the foot of the cross" or something like that, another words God created all of us equal, we may have different talents and abilities that is true, but we are all human beings created equal, each of us having the right to succeed in life on our own terms and live with dignity. No one is better than any one of us and no one is worse than any of us which is a very simple but powerful truth. My own beliefs and perceptions about myself have held me back most of my life from being all I want to be and have hindered me from fully moving forward in my life but not anymore! I used to be so terrified of attending meetings or going on job interviews that I would actually have major anxiety attacks days before a meeting or interview was scheduled and needless to say these situations did not go very well because I was so full of fear and anxiety by the time I got there it turned out to be a great big waste of time because not much can be accomplished in that frame of mind.

The Power of True Self Confidence

Our beliefs about ourselves cause us to walk a certain way and talk a certain way and carry ourselves in a certain way. Our beliefs cause us to give off a silent essence of who we are and how we feel about ourselves whether we realize it or not. My brother has said to me many times "if you don't believe in yourself then no one else will either" and that is so true. Our beliefs about ourselves show whether we realize it or not and people are able to perceive how we feel about ourselves.

I have seen this in my own life and when I started to realize my true value and that I really am equal to other people and not lower than other people I started feeling more confident about myself and believing in myself and when it started sinking deep down into my heart I actually started to carry myself differently. I started walking taller and my posture improved not because I cared about my posture but because the outside of myself was reflecting who I truly was on the inside and people started treating me differently me and showing me more respect because they just sensed the self confidence that I had. I don't understand it but this self confidence carries a silent strength and people can just sense it, it is truly amazing. What was also amazing was the difference of how others treated me when I did not have self confidence or self esteem they sensed that too and they treated me exactly how I felt about myself. I can't explain it but people can just sense the type of person you are and once they sense or perceive how you feel about yourself by the way you carry yourself and the presence that you possess due to your belief system it will determine exactly how they will treat you.

People can just sense that scent of self assurance and self confidence and they take their cue from you as to how they will treat you. So if you have low self esteem and low self confidence people will smell that as well and I am sorry to say but they will just walk all over you and disrespect you and that's just the way it is. Your self esteem and self confidence carry that presence, that weight of self assurance which is easily understood and perceived by others.

I no longer fear what other people think about me because I have come to understand my true value and that I am equal to everyone else. I don't mean that in a rude or arrogant way, what I am saying is that my life's mission is to move forward and accomplish what ever it is that I have been placed on this earth for, it is not to stumble or get side tracked with the opinions of others because I need to say focused on my life, my goals and my responsibilities and the Lord will take care of the rest. I believe what God has said about all of us in the Bible and what He thinks and feels about all the human beings. God has created us and He is the one who as stated in *Jeremiah 29:11(Chapter 29, verse 7) "God promises us a good hope and a good future"* because He loves us and He has placed great values on us. So if God feels that way about us, we should also feel that way about ourselves also, right!

I truly believe that the combination of practicing your speaking skills and developing healthy self esteem and healthy self confidence are the real keys to overcoming your fears of public speaking and becoming a more confident and successful person in life. I don't personally believe that practicing your speaking skills alone is enough to "Permanently Cure your Fear of Public Speaking" because you can practice and practice and practice but if you have not developed true self esteem and true self confidence and have not learned not to fear what other people think of you, you will get up to speak and still be fearful and nervous and anxious because you have not dealt with the source of your public speaking fears which are basically your poor self image and faulty perceptions of yourself whatever they may be, and only you can figure out what those things are.

In life you must be able to speak well or you will never gain the respect and confidence from others that you deserve and you will never be able to speak well until your perceptions about yourself change. Remember if you can't gain the respect and confidence of others, job interviews will never become job offers and business meetings will go no further than just mere meetings. There is great power in self esteem and self confidence and even the Bible says so in *Proverbs 23:7 (Chapter 23, verse 7)* "As a man thinks in his heart, so is he". The Bible states how important it is for us to have a healthy belief system about ourselves. If you believe that you are less than everyone else then you will act like you are less than everyone else and you will carry yourself like you are less than everyone else and you will never move forward in your life because you will think "why should I bother, I'll never be as successful as other people" and that is just not true. The bottom line is that if you believe you have no value you will act like you have no value and you will never reach your full potential in this life. You can be as successful as you want to be in life and accomplish your goals and dreams and do what you enjoy and as my brother has said again "the only one stopping you is you". Oh and by the way I quote my brother several times in this book because he has always given me great advice over the years full of practical wisdom and encouragement and when he has given me advice it has always been right on, so listen up people!

One of my favorite quotes is:

> "Self confidence carries conviction; it makes other people believe in us."
>
> —O.S. Marsden

Speaking Skills Are Very Important

The truth is you can have an excellent education and terrific skills and abilities but if you can't speak well or come across in a confident and self assured manner you will not be able to move forward in your career or in your life no matter what you do. Some how human beings seem to equate speaking well with intelligence so basically even if your skills and abilities are no better than others, if you can speak with confidence and be comfortable in meetings and if you are able to make presentations you will be looked upon differently. I have seen it over and over again and so have many of you, leaders and managers are not better than anyone else and they are generally not more qualified that anyone else, they are just more confident and they are able to speak well in front of others and that makes all the difference in the world my friends.

The truth is that most people sitting in meetings are generally nervous and uncomfortable in some way and you can see it in their eyes and in the way they carry themselves even though they will never admit it. God knows that we fear man because it is just part of our human nature otherwise He would have not put it in the Bible. Most people are fearful and anxious because in their own way they have put on some type of façade, some type of false front for their co-workers and bosses. They are working so hard to try to prove somehow that they have it all together but they don't, which is why I said earlier that behavior modification and techniques will not cause you to win this battle and conquer your public speaking fears. You must first of all be comfortable with just being who you are in front of others, yes just being yourself! So simple but yet so liberating, not trying to put on some type of outward appearance to look good in front of others but just being who you truly are is enough. Being yourself is just the peaceful and quiet knowing of your true value in your heart and that you have nothing to prove to anyone and that you are as equally important and valuable as everyone else in the world and therefore you have nothing to fear, you can just rest in this knowledge once you understand it and apply it to your life. Most people sitting in meetings are not even paying attention to you and what you are saying anyway, they are too busy trying to calm their own fears and insecurities and trying to figure out what they will say if called upon to participate.

Beliefs, Thoughts, Choices

Your beliefs and thoughts about yourself will determine every choice that you make in life so if you suffer with low self esteem and low self confidence it has affected every area of your life whether you want to admit it or not and it will continue to do so until you decide that you want to change and rid yourself of the beliefs that you have about yourself that are holding you back from accomplishing your goals and causing you fear when you speak in public. You will never live up to your full potential and be everything you desire to be in this life until you come to realize that you have great value and worth and that your life counts no matter how bad your life has been up until this point. If you can't believe that right now that's ok too but you can just simply ask God to help you believe that and to save you and help you to know that He has created all of us with great care and infinite wisdom for His glory and the He wants you to succeed and reach your full potential in this life. That in my opinion is true success reaching your full potential as a human being and being all you can be in this life and knowing the God who created you for success and in my opinion there is no higher calling than that. When I say success I don't mean that we will all be millionaires or something like that making lots of money, what I mean is the success of growing and learning and reaching your full potential as a human being and accomplishing the goals and dreams that you have for your life and really feeling good about yourself and being genuinely content with who you are and that in my opinion is true success and by the way, this type of success will build your self esteem and will help you to know your true value and will enable you to able to speak without fear because you will come to understand that you are of equal value and of equal importance as others.

Seeing Yourself as Lower than Other People

I truly believe that the root of all public speaking fears is seeing yourself as less than other people and seeing other people as better than yourself and fearing what these people that you perceive as better than yourself will think about you. We are all members of the human race and we all share the same humanity, we all have the same needs, we need to eat, sleep, go to the bathroom, shower, brush our teeth and go to work, etc. You get the point that I am trying to make, right? You need to see that we are all the same so stop looking at people's outward appearances and start seeing yourself as equal to those whom you view as higher than yourself. You need to see that we are all of equal value. While it is true that we must respect others and be kind to our fellow man, we must also see that our fellow man is just like we are no matter how much money he or she makes, no matter what his or her title is in the company, no matter how educated. The problem is this whole world system has taught us that success and value come from what we look like on the outside or the material things we possess but that is just a lie. We have all been so conditioned to perceive ourselves and others by external things and outward appearances that our society has become extremely shallow and superficial putting on attitudes and heirs to try to impress others and it is very sick. So step out of this foolish and empty way of life and live in the truth. True success is reaching our full potential in life and growing and learning and enjoying life on our own terms and you are the only one that can define what true success means for you. As long as your definition of success is legal and moral and honorable and doesn't hurt anyone and you wouldn't be embarrassed or ashamed to tell your Rabbi, Pastor, Priest, Clergy or mom about it, then go for it!!!

What Are You Believing?

If you are experiencing fear or anxiety about public speaking situations, stop and ask yourself at that very moment what you are believing about yourself that has caused your self esteem and self confidence to drop to such a low level? Are you believing that the people you will be speaking to or meeting with are better than you are? Are you worried or fearful of what they might think of you? Are you believing that you are less or somehow lower than they are? Asking yourself these questions will help you to identify and correct these unhealthy beliefs and will also help you regain your composure if you have allowed your mind and emotions to run away with you and cause you fear and anxiety in a public speaking situation. As you keep practicing these truths while at the same time reinforcing the truth about your true value, eventually it will become very natural to you and you will learn how to replace your unhealthy beliefs and perceptions with the truth about your true value as a human being and this will build your self confidence and self esteem into a solid foundation to build your life and identity upon.

Remember, you have the power to choose what you will believe about yourself and these beliefs must go much deeper than just thoughts about yourself. You must truly believe in your heart that you are valuable not because of what you do for a living or your title or accomplishments but because you are a human being created by God to succeed in life. God loves us and has created us for His own special purposes so that we could reach our full potential as human beings and fulfill our destiny in life, so whether you believe in God or not does not change this fact. God loves us and gave Jesus to take the punishment for our sins that we deserved, so that we would not have to pay it ourselves by spending eternity in hell. The Bible says in *John 15:13 "(Chapter 15, Verse 13) Jesus said, "Greater love hath no man than this that a man lay down his life for his friends"* Jesus gave his life for all of us by being nailed to a cross in order to pay a debt we could never pay for our sins. Jesus has taken the punishment for our sins so that we could go to heaven when we die. We may not have many people in our lives that love us but Jesus loves us and in the book of *Hebrews 13:5-6 (Chapter 13, Verse 5-6) it states that "...Jesus will never leave us or forsake us".* People will always disappoint us in some way but God loves us and has clearly showed us how much He loves and values us by what he has done for us by sending Jesus for us to pay for our sins and show us a better way of life. He has placed great value on all human beings because the Bible says in *1 John 4:16 "God is love".* He loves us and He created us, we are not some freak accident of nature that evolved out of some type of green slime or worms or something. God has carefully handcrafted each one of us for His purpose and for His Glory and He promises us a good future and hope. God promises us a life of peace and dignity and respect and He also accepts us just as we are and therefore we can be comfortable and content with who we are and we don't have to try to be something that we're not. *Our Declaration of Independence written July 4, 1776 states "We hold these truths to be self evident; that all men are created equal and endowed by their Creator with certain unalienable rights and among these are life, liberty and the pursuit of happiness".*

We Have Choices

We have no control over other people or how they choose to treat us but we do have control over how we perceive the treatment of others and how we allow the treatment of others to affect us. When I was a very young child I did not have the ability to choose how I perceived the beatings I received by my father, I was not able to understand at that time that I was not a worthless piece of garbage and that I was not to blame for my dad's alcohol problems and the beatings I received. My dad was the one who had the lifelong drinking problem and took out his anger on my brother and I with "the strap". But now as an adult I do understand that my parent's divorce and the beatings I received were not my fault and that I do have value and that I am a very capable and worthwhile person with goals and dreams. So my point is that we all have a choice of how we will perceive the treatment of others and what we choose to believe about ourselves. We should no longer interpret that the poor treatment we receive from others means that we have no value or that we have less value than they have. They are the one's that have the problem not us. We don't have to allow situations or people's treatment of us to determine or define our value or to cause us to have low self esteem and low self confidence. We must choose how we will interpret our interactions with people. It is only when we start taking responsibility for our beliefs and perceptions of ourselves and others that we can truly experience peace and joy and contentment with just being ourselves and then we will finally be free of fear and anxiety when we have to speak in public.

Life Changing Truths

My life has truly been changed and has opened up to me in new and different ways. I am now able to see great possibilities instead of limitations. I am now able to see that I have choices and that if I don't like something I can change it. I have the power to choose the direction I want my life to go in. Life seems a lot brighter now not only because of my faith in God but because I am also confident in myself and it feels good. I no longer want to avoid public speaking situations because I don't care anymore about what other people think about me and I am not afraid to just be myself. I am not afraid to make mistakes and I am not afraid of making mistakes in front of others. Life is too short so don't be afraid to step out of your comfort zone and overcome your public speaking fears by developing true and healthy beliefs and perceptions about yourself because in doing so you will be transformed and your self esteem and self confidence will grow and then you will be able to stand up and speak without fear to anyone or any audience at any time not because you are the best speaker in the world but because you know your true value and knowing your true value is the real key to conquering all of the fears and anxieties that you have about public speaking. Knowing your true value is really the key to building and developing healthy self esteem and healthy self confidence and it is this healthy belief system that will just naturally cause you to become a more confident and fearless speaker. I might even dare to say that you are probably a great speaker already you just have lots of faulty perceptions and unhealthy beliefs that have covered up and hindered your true speaking ability. But as I have said many times throughout this book and I think it is worth repeating, I believe that the fears, anxieties and phobias of public speaking that I have faced and that each of you are facing to one degree or another are just the results of the real issues of low self esteem, low self confidence and fearing what others think about us. See for yourself, start to develop real and genuine self esteem and self confidence and see if you don't automatically become a better speaker and a much more confident person not only in public speaking situations and social situations but in life in general. I think you will all be pleasantly surprised as you deal with your own negative perceptions in certain areas of your lives that are causing you fears and anxieties of speaking to an audience that you will naturally become more comfortable with speaking in public, it will just be a natural and automatic result of the healthy beliefs that you are developing about yourself.

My goal is not to become the most talented and gifted speaker on the planet because I certainly am not but my goal and the goal of this book is to just encourage you to be the best speaker that you can be, not comparing yourself to others and their speaking styles but comparing yourself with yourself. Compare yourself with where you are now to a future point in time so you can see your growth and progress and then you will become encouraged as you take this journey to help yourself overcome your faulty beliefs which cause you to fear speaking in public and you will be proud of how much more comfortable you are in speaking in front of a group compared to what you used to be like.

The object of this book is to provide you with some insight into some of the things that I have learned about myself from my own battle with the fear of public speaking and I believe these things will help you to help yourself with whatever type of speaking you must do in your life. Whether it be a job interview or making a presentation to a group, or social gatherings, the more comfortable you are in speaking to individuals or groups will be in direct proportion to the level of self esteem and self confidence you develop. You must create a healthy and true belief system about yourself in order to overcome your fear of public speaking. I encourage you to learn not to fear what other people think of you and not to try to make a good impression or to look good in front of others but to just be yourself because that is truly enough. Step off the merry go round of trying to always please others or impress others because it really doesn't matter what people think about you and it is these types of things that have probably caused most of us great fear and anxiety in public speaking situations anyway.

Genuine and True Self Esteem and Self Confidence

When you develop true and healthy self esteem and self confidence you won't care about what other people think about you because you will finally be free to be who you really are and live and enjoy your life. Who knows some of you may well become very accomplished speakers, some of you may need help just sharing your opinions at the next PTA meeting or homeowners association meeting but whatever your public speaking needs are if you have a healthy belief system you will be able to speak without fear anywhere and at any time and that is the bottom line. As you take this journey to help yourself overcome your fears of public speaking I believe that you will see yourself becoming a more confident and assertive person not in an ugly or obnoxious way but in an honorable and dignified way knowing that what you have to say is as equally important as those who seem to love the spotlight, you know those same people that must constantly make their thoughts and opinions known at every meeting or gathering, you know those that when they start speaking you just roll your eyes and say "here we go again", well here's a newsflash for you, the things you want to share or speak about are of equal value and importance to those who think that they are the only ones that could possibly have anything intelligent to say.

As I mentioned earlier you probably already are a good speaker but you just have all of these hang ups and insecurities about yourself that cover up the real you which causes you a lot of fear and anxiety about public speaking. I don't think anyone really has the fear of public speaking, what I believe is that each of us has our own unique set of hang ups and fears and insecurities about ourselves and because of these things we fear facing an audience. Conquering your low self esteem and poor self image is a process of learning but I don't believe it will take very long at all as long as you make the commitment to yourself to change your beliefs, opinions and perceptions about yourself and put what you have learned into practice.

I mentioned earlier that techniques and gimmicks are not going to give you the real results you are looking for. There are plenty of seminars, books and tapes out there that claim to have the best tips and techniques for your public speaking fears but genuine and permanent change must come from within you, it is not something that you can just apply externally like a bandage.

I have seen many people that from all outward appearances look like they have "made it". The right cars, the big house, the right job and even the right plastic surgeon and from the outside it looks like these people have really become great successes in life. While it is true that each of us has the right to define what success means to us personally, most outwardly successful people are very insecure and have very low self esteem and self confidence because they have been trying to buy it or acquire it somehow, but true and genuine self esteem and self confidence do not come from anything that you own or accomplish, plain and simple. True self esteem and true self confidence come from knowing that you are a valuable human being at the very core of who you are with nothing else added.

There are plenty of resources in the world to help you create a healthy belief system based upon the true principles of just being a human being. I personally use the Bible as my guide for life and my belief system because of the time tested truths about God, our world and the human race He created. The Bible has sold more copies than any other book in history and is still a bestseller today. The bottom line is that all of these passing fads and temporary pursuits in life will leave us empty and feeling worthless and dry but God's word the Bible fills us up each and every time we read it. It renews our hope, gives us inner strength, builds our faith, gives us the wisdom and strength that we need for each day and promises us eternal security and a clear explanation of what will happen to us when we die. It tells us who God is and why He created us and it tells us how much we mean to Him and how much He values us and that is exactly what those of us with low self esteem and low self confidence need to know, our value. Once you rid yourself of the faulty beliefs and perceptions that you have about yourself in the areas that I have described throughout this book is when you will truly be a confident speaker because you will become a more confident person and you will be comfortable and fearless speaking to any type of audience because you won't fear what other people think about you anymore because of what you have learned to think and believe about yourself!

God bless each and every one of you as you attempt to apply these principles and concepts to your lives. I hope to see each one of you standing in front of your own audience one day unafraid to express yourself and to be comfortable in just being yourself finally free and VICTORIOUS!!!!

References

The Holy Bible, Authorized King James Version 1611

The Declaration of Independence

Index

T

thoughts 13, 15, 18, 19, 20, 26, 53, 58, 67
true value 8, 57, 63
truth 16, 41, 44, 46, 51, 56, 57

V

value 7, 9, 10, 29, 30, 31, 33, 35, 40, 43, 45, 47, 50, 52, 53, 55, 57, 58, 61, 63, 68, 69

Breinigsville, PA USA
22 December 2009
229643BV00001B/11/A